Chapter 1: Introduction to Diabetes Insipidus

Understanding Diabetes Insipidus

Diabetes insipidus (DI) is a rare condition characterized by an imbalance of fluids in the body, leading to excessive thirst and frequent urination. Unlike diabetes mellitus, which involves issues with insulin and blood sugar levels, diabetes insipidus primarily stems from problems with the hormone vasopressin, also known as antidiuretic hormone (ADH). This hormone plays a crucial role in regulating the body's water balance by signaling the kidneys to reabsorb water. When there is insufficient production of vasopressin or the body becomes resistant to its effects, it results in the inability to concentrate urine, thereby causing the symptoms associated with DI.

There are several causes of diabetes insipidus, which can be broadly categorized into central and nephrogenic types. Central diabetes insipidus occurs when there is damage to the hypothalamus or pituitary gland, often due to trauma, surgery, tumors, or conditions like autoimmune diseases. Nephrogenic diabetes insipidus, on the other hand, arises when the kidneys fail to respond to vasopressin. This can result from genetic factors, chronic kidney disease, or the effects of certain medications. Understanding these distinctions is essential for both patients and healthcare providers to determine the appropriate course of action.

Diagnosis of diabetes insipidus typically involves a combination of patient history, physical examinations, and specific tests. Initial assessments may include a water deprivation test, which measures how the body responds to dehydration, and a vasopressin stimulation test, which evaluates how well the kidneys respond to ADH. Other diagnostic tools may involve blood tests to check electrolyte levels and urine tests to assess concentration. Accurate diagnosis is vital, as it helps differentiate DI from other conditions that present similar symptoms, such as diabetes mellitus or urinary tract infections.

Treatment options for diabetes insipidus primarily focus on managing symptoms and restoring fluid balance. For central diabetes insipidus, desmopressin, a synthetic form of vasopressin, is often prescribed to help reduce urine output and alleviate thirst. In cases of nephrogenic diabetes insipidus, treatment may involve addressing the underlying cause, modifying medications that contribute to the condition, or using diuretics to help control symptoms. Lifestyle changes, such as increasing fluid intake and adjusting diet to include foods with higher water content, also play a critical role in managing the condition effectively.

Living with diabetes insipidus can have psychological implications, as patients may experience anxiety or frustration related to their symptoms and the constant need for hydration. Support systems, including counseling and support groups, can be beneficial in helping individuals cope with the emotional challenges associated with the condition. For caregivers, understanding the complexities of diabetes insipidus is essential for providing effective support and managing the daily challenges faced by the patient. Through education and proactive management strategies, both patients and caregivers can work together to navigate the intricacies of living with diabetes insipidus, ensuring a better quality of life.

Types of Diabetes Insipidus

Diabetes insipidus is a rare condition characterized by excessive thirst and the production of large amounts of dilute urine. Understanding the types of diabetes insipidus is crucial for patients, as it can influence diagnosis, management, and treatment options. The two main types are central diabetes insipidus and nephrogenic diabetes insipidus. Each type has distinct underlying causes, symptoms, and approaches to treatment, making it essential for patients to recognize these differences.

Central diabetes insipidus occurs when the body does not produce enough of the hormone vasopressin, also known as antidiuretic hormone (ADH). This hormone is produced in the hypothalamus and stored in the pituitary gland. A deficiency in vasopressin can result from various factors, including head injuries, tumors, or genetic disorders. Patients may experience intense thirst and frequent urination, as the kidneys cannot retain water without adequate levels of this hormone. Treatment often involves hormone replacement therapy, which can help manage symptoms effectively and restore a more normal urinary pattern.

Nephrogenic diabetes insipidus, on the other hand, is caused by the kidneys' inability to respond to vasopressin. In this case, the hormone is produced in normal amounts, but the kidneys fail to reabsorb water properly. This condition can be inherited or acquired, with potential causes including chronic kidney disease, certain medications, or electrolyte imbalances, particularly high levels of calcium. Patients with nephrogenic diabetes insipidus also present with similar symptoms of excessive thirst and urination, but their treatment may focus on addressing the underlying causes, adjusting medication, or implementing dietary changes to help manage fluid balance.

There is also a third, less common type known as dipsogenic diabetes insipidus, which arises from an abnormal thirst mechanism in the hypothalamus. Individuals with this type may drink excessive amounts of water, leading to a dilution of blood sodium levels and resulting in symptoms similar to those of central diabetes insipidus. This form is often linked to psychological conditions or can occur following certain brain injuries. Management of dipsogenic diabetes insipidus typically involves behavioral strategies and monitoring fluid intake to prevent complications.

Understanding the different types of diabetes insipidus is essential for patients, as it guides the path to appropriate diagnosis and treatment. Each type has unique characteristics and management strategies, and recognizing these differences can empower patients in their healthcare journey. By working closely with healthcare providers, patients can develop personalized treatment plans that address their specific needs and improve their quality of life.

Importance of Awareness

Awareness of diabetes insipidus is crucial for patients and their families, as it plays a significant role in managing this condition effectively. Understanding the nuances of diabetes insipidus, including its causes and risk factors, empowers patients to recognize symptoms early and seek appropriate medical attention. This proactive approach can prevent complications and improve overall quality of life. By being informed, patients can participate actively in discussions with healthcare providers, ensuring that their concerns are addressed and that they receive tailored treatment options.

Knowledge about the diagnostic process is another critical aspect of awareness. Patients should be educated on the various testing methods used to diagnose diabetes insipidus, such as water deprivation tests and urine concentration tests. Being aware of these methods not only alleviates anxiety associated with medical procedures but also helps patients understand the rationale behind their healthcare provider's recommendations. This understanding fosters a sense of control over their health journey, encouraging patients to ask questions and engage in their treatment plan.

Awareness extends beyond the clinical aspects of diabetes insipidus; it includes recognizing the lifestyle changes necessary for effective management. Patients need to understand the importance of hydration, dietary considerations, and medication adherence. By adapting their daily routines to accommodate their condition, they can significantly mitigate symptoms and enhance their well-being. Furthermore, cultivating a support network of family and friends who understand diabetes insipidus can provide emotional support and practical assistance, making the management process less isolating.

The psychological impact of living with diabetes insipidus is another vital area of awareness. Patients may experience feelings of frustration, anxiety, or depression due to the unpredictable nature of their symptoms. Understanding that these feelings are common can help patients cope better and seek support when necessary. Mental health resources, including counseling or support groups, can be beneficial for addressing these challenges. Awareness of the psychological aspects of the condition allows patients to approach their health holistically, considering both physical and emotional well-being.

Lastly, awareness of potential complications and long-term effects associated with diabetes insipidus is essential for patient education. Understanding risks such as kidney damage or electrolyte imbalances can motivate patients to adhere to their treatment plans and make necessary lifestyle adjustments. This comprehensive awareness not only prepares patients for the challenges they may face but also empowers them to take charge of their health. Ultimately, informed patients are better equipped to navigate the complexities of diabetes insipidus, leading to more effective management and improved outcomes.

Chapter 2: Causes of Diabetes Insipidus

Central Diabetes Insipidus

Central Diabetes Insipidus (CDI) is a type of diabetes insipidus characterized by a deficiency of the hormone vasopressin, also known as antidiuretic hormone (ADH). This hormone is produced in the hypothalamus and stored in the pituitary gland, playing a crucial role in regulating the body's fluid balance. In patients with CDI, the lack of vasopressin leads to excessive urination and increased thirst, as the kidneys cannot concentrate urine effectively. Understanding the underlying causes of CDI is essential for patients to manage their condition effectively.

The primary cause of central diabetes insipidus is damage to the hypothalamus or pituitary gland, which can occur due to various factors. This damage may result from head trauma, surgical procedures, tumors, or infections that affect the brain. Additionally, autoimmunity can lead to the destruction of the cells that produce vasopressin. In some cases, the cause remains idiopathic, meaning that it is unknown. Recognizing these causes is crucial for patients and healthcare providers, as they can influence treatment decisions and management strategies.

Diagnosis of central diabetes insipidus typically involves a combination of clinical evaluation and specific tests. Patients often present with symptoms such as polyuria (excessive urination) and polydipsia (excessive thirst). Healthcare providers may conduct a water deprivation test to assess the body's ability to concentrate urine and determine the presence of CDI. Other diagnostic tools include MRI scans to visualize the pituitary gland and rule out potential tumors or structural abnormalities. Understanding the diagnostic process can help patients feel more empowered and informed about their condition.

Treatment options for central diabetes insipidus primarily focus on replacing the missing hormone. Desmopressin, a synthetic form of vasopressin, is commonly prescribed and can be administered as a nasal spray or oral tablet. This medication helps to reduce urine output and alleviate symptoms of excessive thirst. In some cases, addressing underlying causes, such as treating a tumor or managing an autoimmune condition, may also be necessary. Patients should discuss potential side effects and the need for ongoing monitoring with their healthcare provider to ensure effective management of their condition.

Living with central diabetes insipidus requires significant lifestyle adjustments to maintain health and comfort. Patients are encouraged to establish a routine for fluid intake, ensuring they stay adequately hydrated while managing their symptoms. It is essential to monitor urine output and recognize signs of dehydration. Psychological support is also vital, as managing a chronic condition can impact mental health. Joining support groups or seeking counseling can help patients and their caregivers cope with the emotional challenges of living with diabetes insipidus, fostering a sense of community and shared understanding.

Nephrogenic Diabetes Insipidus

Nephrogenic diabetes insipidus (NDI) is a condition characterized by the kidneys' inability to respond to the hormone vasopressin, also known as antidiuretic hormone (ADH). This results in the kidneys being unable to concentrate urine, leading to excessive urination and thirst. Unlike central diabetes insipidus, where the problem lies in insufficient production of ADH, nephrogenic diabetes insipidus stems from a defect in the kidney tubules. This condition can be acquired or inherited and is essential for patients to understand due to its implications on management and lifestyle.

The causes of nephrogenic diabetes insipidus can vary significantly. Genetic mutations, particularly in the AVPR2 gene, can lead to the inherited form of the condition, primarily affecting males. Acquired NDI can result from various factors, including chronic kidney disease, certain medications such as lithium, and electrolyte imbalances, particularly hypercalcemia and hypokalemia. Understanding these causes is vital for patients as it helps identify potential risk factors and informs decisions regarding treatment and lifestyle adjustments.

Diagnosing nephrogenic diabetes insipidus typically involves a combination of clinical evaluation and specific testing methods. Patients usually present with symptoms such as polyuria (excessive urination) and polydipsia (excessive thirst). A water deprivation test, which assesses the kidneys' ability to concentrate urine, is often conducted to differentiate between types of diabetes insipidus. Blood and urine tests may also be performed to check for electrolyte levels and kidney function. Accurate diagnosis is crucial, as it influences the management strategies employed.

Treatment options for nephrogenic diabetes insipidus focus on addressing the underlying cause, if possible, and managing symptoms. In cases linked to medications, adjusting or discontinuing the offending drug may alleviate symptoms. Thiazide diuretics, despite their function, paradoxically reduce urine output in some patients with NDI. Additionally, a low-salt diet can help minimize urine output by reducing the kidneys' burden. Patients are encouraged to maintain adequate hydration, as the body struggles to retain water.

Living with nephrogenic diabetes insipidus requires several lifestyle changes to manage the condition effectively. Patients should be vigilant about their fluid intake and may need to carry water at all times to avoid dehydration. Monitoring urine output can help in recognizing any changes in the condition. Regular follow-ups with healthcare providers are essential to adjust treatment as necessary and to screen for potential complications. By understanding nephrogenic diabetes insipidus and adopting proactive management strategies, patients can enhance their quality of life and mitigate the challenges posed by this condition.

Dipsogenic Diabetes Insipidus

Dipsogenic diabetes insipidus is a specific form of diabetes insipidus characterized by excessive fluid intake, leading to an increased need for urination. This condition arises due to a dysfunction in the mechanisms that regulate thirst, often triggered by damage to the hypothalamus or the pituitary gland. Unlike the more common forms of diabetes insipidus, which are primarily related to a deficiency of the hormone vasopressin, dipsogenic diabetes insipidus is associated with the patient's behavior, particularly in the context of excessive drinking. Understanding the underlying causes and recognizing the symptoms is essential for effective management and treatment.

The primary cause of dipsogenic diabetes insipidus is often linked to psychological factors or damage to the hypothalamus. Individuals with certain psychiatric conditions may develop a compulsive need to drink large amounts of water, leading to a state of chronic overhydration. Additionally, physical damage to the hypothalamus, perhaps due to trauma, tumors, or surgical interventions, can disrupt normal thirst regulation. It is crucial for patients to understand these risk factors, as they can influence both the diagnosis and the approach to treatment.

Diagnosing dipsogenic diabetes insipidus involves a detailed medical history and a series of tests to evaluate urine output and thirst response. A water deprivation test is commonly used to differentiate between central diabetes insipidus, nephrogenic diabetes insipidus, and dipsogenic diabetes insipidus. This test measures how well the body can concentrate urine when fluid intake is restricted. Patients may also undergo imaging studies to assess any structural abnormalities in the hypothalamus or pituitary gland, which could contribute to the condition.

Treatment options for dipsogenic diabetes insipidus primarily focus on managing fluid intake and addressing any underlying psychological issues. Behavioral therapy may be beneficial for patients who exhibit compulsive drinking behaviors. In some cases, medications that help regulate thirst or manage associated psychiatric conditions may be prescribed. Additionally, education on the importance of hydration without overconsumption is vital.

Patients should work closely with their healthcare team to develop a tailored approach that considers their individual needs and circumstances.

Living with dipsogenic diabetes insipidus can have psychological impacts, particularly related to the constant need for urination and the challenges of managing fluid intake. Patients may experience anxiety or embarrassment in social situations due to their condition. Support groups or counseling may be beneficial in helping patients cope with these feelings. Furthermore, caregivers play a crucial role in providing support, understanding, and encouragement as patients navigate the complexities of their condition. Establishing a routine for monitoring fluid intake and maintaining open communication with healthcare providers can also enhance management strategies and overall quality of life.

Gestational Diabetes Insipidus

Gestational diabetes insipidus is a rare form of diabetes insipidus that occurs during pregnancy. It is characterized by an inability of the body to properly regulate water balance, leading to excessive thirst and urination. While diabetes insipidus is primarily understood as a condition linked to deficiencies in the hormone vasopressin, gestational diabetes insipidus typically arises due to hormonal changes during pregnancy that affect the body's ability to respond to this hormone. This condition may be temporary and often resolves after childbirth, but understanding its mechanisms and implications is important for those affected.

The causes of gestational diabetes insipidus involve the interplay of various hormones that fluctuate during pregnancy. Notably, the placenta produces a hormone called placental vasopressinase, which can break down vasopressin, leading to lower levels of this hormone in the bloodstream. This reduction can disrupt the normal balance of fluids in the body, resulting in the classic symptoms of diabetes insipidus. Additionally, pregnancy-related changes in kidney function and fluid balance can contribute to the onset of this condition, making it crucial for pregnant individuals to be aware of the signs and symptoms.

Diagnosis of gestational diabetes insipidus typically involves a thorough assessment of a patient's medical history, symptoms, and laboratory tests. Healthcare providers may perform a water deprivation test to determine the body's ability to concentrate urine, along with measuring levels of vasopressin. It is also important to rule out other forms of diabetes insipidus or conditions that may mimic its symptoms. Accurate diagnosis is essential, as it informs the appropriate management strategies and helps in monitoring the health of both the mother and the developing fetus.

Treatment options for gestational diabetes insipidus focus on managing symptoms and ensuring the health of both the mother and the baby. In many cases, the condition may not require specific medical intervention, as symptoms often improve after delivery. However, for those experiencing significant discomfort or health risks, medications such as desmopressin may be prescribed to help manage symptoms by mimicking the action of vasopressin. Close monitoring by healthcare professionals is essential to adapt treatment plans as necessary throughout the pregnancy.

Living with gestational diabetes insipidus can pose unique challenges, particularly as it relates to lifestyle and emotional well-being. Patients are encouraged to stay well-hydrated and to monitor their symptoms regularly. Support from healthcare providers, family, and counseling services can help manage the psychological impact of the condition. Additionally, understanding dietary considerations and making appropriate lifestyle changes can contribute to a more comfortable pregnancy experience. With effective management, most individuals can navigate gestational diabetes insipidus successfully and focus on the joy of motherhood.

Chapter 3: Risk Factors for Diabetes Insipidus

Genetic Factors

Genetic factors play a significant role in the development of diabetes insipidus, influencing both its occurrence and progression. While the condition may arise sporadically, certain hereditary patterns have been identified, particularly in cases of nephrogenic diabetes insipidus. This form occurs when the kidneys are unable to respond to antidiuretic hormone (ADH) due to genetic mutations. These mutations often affect the aquaporin-2 gene, essential for water reabsorption in the kidneys, leading to excessive urination and thirst. Understanding these genetic predispositions can help patients and their families navigate the complexities of this condition.

In addition to nephrogenic diabetes insipidus, central diabetes insipidus can also have genetic underpinnings, though it is more commonly acquired through trauma, tumors, or diseases affecting the pituitary gland. Some rare genetic syndromes have been associated with central diabetes insipidus, including Wolfram syndrome and Laurence-Moon-Biedl syndrome. Identifying these connections can be crucial for patients, as it may guide both diagnosis and management strategies. Genetic counseling can provide valuable insights for families with a history of diabetes insipidus, enabling them to understand their risks and make informed decisions regarding testing and treatment.

Genetic testing can be an important tool in diagnosing diabetes insipidus, particularly when a hereditary component is suspected. For families with a known history of genetic mutations linked to the condition, proactive testing can help identify at-risk individuals early. This approach not only aids in timely intervention but also assists in the monitoring of symptoms and potential complications. Patients should discuss the possibility of genetic testing with their healthcare provider, especially if they have a family history or experience unexplained symptoms.

Understanding the genetic factors associated with diabetes insipidus can also enhance treatment options. For those diagnosed with nephrogenic diabetes insipidus due to genetic mutations, certain medications may be more effective based on the specific mutation present. In some cases, lifestyle modifications and dietary adjustments may further aid in managing symptoms, while genetic insights can help tailor approaches to hydration and electrolyte balance. Engaging with healthcare providers about genetic implications can empower patients to take an active role in their treatment plans.

Finally, the psychological impact of knowing one's genetic predisposition to diabetes insipidus cannot be overlooked. Patients may experience anxiety or uncertainty about their condition and its management. By fostering open communication with healthcare professionals and support networks, patients can find reassurance and guidance as they navigate their diagnosis. Awareness and understanding of genetic factors in diabetes insipidus not only foster better management strategies but also cultivate a sense of agency and community among those affected by this condition.

Medical Conditions

Medical conditions associated with diabetes insipidus can significantly impact a patient's quality of life. Diabetes insipidus itself is characterized by an imbalance of fluids in the body, leading to excessive thirst and urination. This condition arises when the body does not produce sufficient amounts of the antidiuretic hormone (ADH), also known as vasopressin, or when the kidneys are unable to respond to this hormone effectively. Understanding the underlying causes of diabetes insipidus is crucial, as it can help patients and healthcare providers identify potential complications and develop appropriate management strategies.

There are two primary types of diabetes insipidus: central and nephrogenic. Central diabetes insipidus occurs when the hypothalamus or pituitary gland is damaged, leading to decreased secretion of ADH. This damage can result from various medical conditions, including head injuries, brain tumors, or infections affecting the brain. On the other hand, nephrogenic diabetes insipidus is caused by the kidneys' inability to respond to ADH, often due to genetic factors or chronic kidney disease. Identifying the type of diabetes insipidus a patient has is essential for determining the most effective treatment options.

In addition to diabetes insipidus, patients may also experience other medical conditions that can exacerbate their symptoms. For instance, individuals with diabetes insipidus may have a higher risk of dehydration due to the inability to concentrate urine, which can lead to electrolyte imbalances and complications such as kidney damage. Furthermore, conditions that affect fluid balance, such as congestive heart failure or certain endocrine disorders, can complicate the management of diabetes insipidus. Regular monitoring and a comprehensive understanding of these associated conditions are vital for effective patient care.

Diagnosis and testing methods for diabetes insipidus involve a thorough medical history, physical examination, and specific laboratory tests. Healthcare providers may conduct a water deprivation test to assess the body's ability to concentrate urine and evaluate the patient's response to ADH. Additionally, blood tests can help rule out other underlying medical issues that could be contributing to the symptoms. Accurate diagnosis is crucial for implementing the appropriate treatment plan tailored to the patient's unique needs, which may include hormone replacement therapy or other interventions.

Living with diabetes insipidus can pose various lifestyle challenges and psychological impacts. Patients often need to make significant adjustments to their daily routines, including monitoring fluid intake and output. Support from caregivers and healthcare professionals is essential in helping patients cope with the emotional and psychological aspects of the condition. As individuals manage their diabetes insipidus, they should also consider dietary choices that support overall health and hydration, while being aware of potential complications that could arise from this chronic condition. Understanding these medical conditions and their interrelated nature can empower patients to take charge of their health and well-being.

Medications

Medications play a crucial role in the management of diabetes insipidus (DI), a condition characterized by the body's inability to properly regulate water balance due to insufficient production of the hormone vasopressin, also known as antidiuretic hormone (ADH). The primary medication used in the treatment of central diabetes insipidus is desmopressin, a synthetic analog of vasopressin. Desmopressin works by mimicking the action of ADH, promoting water reabsorption in the kidneys and helping to reduce excessive urination and thirst. It is available in various forms, including nasal spray, oral tablets, and injectable solutions, allowing for flexible administration based on patient needs and preferences.

For patients with nephrogenic diabetes insipidus, where the kidneys do not respond to ADH, treatment focuses on addressing the underlying causes, if identifiable. In some cases, diuretics such as hydrochlorothiazide may paradoxically help reduce urine output. This is because thiazide diuretics can promote water reabsorption in the proximal part of the nephron, thereby decreasing the volume of urine produced. Additionally, non-steroidal anti-inflammatory drugs (NSAIDs) may also be prescribed to help manage symptoms, though their effectiveness can vary among individuals.

Monitoring medication effectiveness and side effects is essential for patients managing diabetes insipidus. Regular follow-ups with healthcare providers are necessary to adjust dosages and assess the response to treatment. Patients should be aware of potential side effects associated with desmopressin, which can include headache, nausea, and in rare cases, water retention leading to hyponatremia (low sodium levels). Understanding these risks enables patients to recognize symptoms early and seek prompt medical advice if needed.

Lifestyle modifications can complement medication management for diabetes insipidus. Patients are often encouraged to maintain a fluid intake that matches their output, ensuring adequate hydration. Keeping a daily record of fluid intake and urine output can help both patients and healthcare providers evaluate the effectiveness of treatment and make necessary adjustments. Patients should also be educated about the importance of adhering to their prescribed medication regimen to minimize complications and optimize their quality of life.

In conclusion, while medications are vital in managing diabetes insipidus, they are most effective when combined with lifestyle strategies and regular medical supervision. Patients should actively engage in their treatment plan, communicate openly with their healthcare providers, and educate themselves about their condition. This proactive approach helps improve the management of diabetes insipidus and enhances overall well-being, allowing individuals to lead fulfilling lives despite the challenges posed by this condition.

Lifestyle Factors

Lifestyle factors play a significant role in managing diabetes insipidus and can greatly influence a patient's overall well-being. Understanding how daily habits, routines, and choices impact hydration, health, and the effectiveness of treatment can empower patients to take an active role in their care. By making informed lifestyle changes, individuals can better control their symptoms and improve their quality of life.

One of the most critical lifestyle factors for managing diabetes insipidus is fluid intake. Patients must pay close attention to their hydration levels, often requiring them to drink large amounts of water throughout the day to prevent dehydration. Establishing a consistent routine for fluid intake can be beneficial. Patients are encouraged to carry a water bottle and set reminders to drink regularly, particularly in situations where they may forget, such as during busy workdays or social events. Additionally, understanding the signs of dehydration, such as dry mouth, fatigue, and dizziness, can help patients act quickly to address their hydration needs.

Dietary considerations also play an essential role in the management of diabetes insipidus. While there are no specific dietary restrictions for individuals with this condition, maintaining a balanced diet can support overall health. Incorporating foods with high water content, such as fruits and vegetables, can aid in hydration. Furthermore, reducing the intake of caffeine and alcohol is advisable, as both can have diuretic effects, potentially exacerbating symptoms. Patients should consult with healthcare providers or nutritionists to develop personalized dietary plans that align with their hydration needs and overall health goals.

Physical activity and exercise are additional lifestyle factors that can influence the management of diabetes insipidus. Regular exercise can help improve overall health and may enhance the body's ability to regulate fluids. However, it is crucial for patients to be mindful of their hydration status before, during, and after physical activity. Engaging in moderate exercise, such as walking or swimming, can be beneficial, but patients should avoid intense workouts that could lead to excessive fluid loss without proper hydration management. Listening to one's body and adjusting exercise routines based on individual hydration needs is essential.

Finally, psychological factors should not be overlooked when considering lifestyle changes for managing diabetes insipidus. Living with a chronic condition can bring about feelings of anxiety or frustration, impacting daily life and overall health. Patients are encouraged to seek support from mental health professionals or support groups to address these feelings. Mindfulness practices, such as meditation or yoga, can also be beneficial in managing stress and promoting emotional well-being. By addressing both the physical and psychological aspects of living with diabetes insipidus, patients can develop a more comprehensive approach to their health and improve their overall quality of life.

Chapter 4: Diagnosis and Testing Methods

Initial Assessment

Initial assessment of diabetes insipidus is crucial for determining the appropriate course of action for management and treatment. When a patient presents symptoms such as excessive thirst and increased urination, medical professionals will begin by gathering a comprehensive medical history. This includes asking about the onset, duration, and severity of symptoms, as well as any relevant family history of diabetes insipidus or other endocrine disorders. Understanding these factors helps in identifying potential causes and risk factors associated with the condition.

Physical examinations play an important role in the initial assessment. Healthcare providers will check for signs of dehydration, as this condition often leads to significant fluid loss. They may measure vital signs, including blood pressure and heart rate, to assess the patient's overall state of health. Additionally, examining the skin for signs of dryness or poor turgor can provide valuable information regarding the patient's hydration status. These initial observations can guide further diagnostic testing.

Laboratory tests are essential in confirming a diagnosis of diabetes insipidus. Blood tests may be performed to evaluate electrolyte levels, kidney function, and the concentration of certain hormones. A urine test will typically follow, measuring the concentration of urine to determine its osmolality. In cases where the diagnosis remains uncertain, a water deprivation test may be conducted. This test assesses the body's ability to concentrate urine in the absence of fluid intake, which can help differentiate between central diabetes insipidus and nephrogenic diabetes insipidus.

In addition to laboratory tests, imaging studies such as MRI scans may be utilized to examine the pituitary gland and hypothalamus. These imaging techniques can help identify any structural abnormalities or lesions that might be contributing to the development of diabetes insipidus. The combination of clinical evaluation, laboratory tests, and imaging studies forms a comprehensive approach to accurately diagnosing the condition and understanding its underlying causes.

Understanding the initial assessment process empowers patients to engage actively in their healthcare. Being aware of what to expect during the assessment phase can alleviate anxiety and foster a better patient-provider relationship. By cooperating with medical professionals and providing detailed information about their symptoms, patients can help ensure that the assessment is thorough, leading to timely and effective management of diabetes insipidus.

Urine Tests

Urine tests are an essential diagnostic tool in the evaluation of diabetes insipidus. These tests provide critical information about the kidneys' ability to concentrate urine, which is a key factor in distinguishing diabetes insipidus from other conditions that can cause excessive thirst and urination. Typically, urine tests involve measuring the concentration of solutes in the urine, primarily focusing on specific gravity and osmolality. In patients with diabetes insipidus, urine tends to be dilute, reflecting the kidneys' inability to concentrate urine effectively.

One of the most common urine tests used in the diagnosis of diabetes insipidus is the 24-hour urine collection. During this test, patients are asked to collect all their urine over a 24-hour period. The collected urine is then analyzed for volume and concentration. A high volume of dilute urine is indicative of diabetes insipidus, while normal or concentrated urine may suggest other causes of polyuria, such as diabetes mellitus or certain kidney disorders. This test is often conducted alongside blood tests to provide a comprehensive view of the patient's hydration status and kidney function.

In addition to the 24-hour collection, spot urine tests can also be performed. These tests involve analyzing a single urine sample for specific gravity and osmolality. A low specific gravity (below 1.005) and low urine osmolality (below 300 mOsm/kg) are suggestive of diabetes insipidus. It is important for patients to understand that these tests are typically ordered in conjunction with other diagnostic procedures, such as water deprivation tests, which help to further differentiate between central diabetes insipidus and nephrogenic diabetes insipidus.

Patients should be aware that hydration status can significantly affect urine test results. It is essential to follow the healthcare provider's instructions regarding fluid intake before these tests. For instance, during the water deprivation test, patients may be asked to restrict fluid intake for a certain period to assess their body's response to dehydration. This test helps determine the underlying cause of diabetes insipidus by evaluating how well the kidneys concentrate urine when fluid intake is limited.

Ultimately, urine tests play a crucial role in the diagnosis and management of diabetes insipidus. Understanding the significance of these tests can empower patients to actively engage in their care. By being informed about the testing process and its implications, patients can better communicate with their healthcare providers, leading to timely diagnosis and appropriate treatment options tailored to their specific needs.

Blood Tests

Blood tests play a crucial role in the diagnosis and management of diabetes insipidus. When a patient presents symptoms such as excessive thirst and frequent urination, healthcare providers often begin their evaluation with a comprehensive blood test. These tests help assess kidney function, electrolyte levels, and the presence of other conditions that may mimic or contribute to the symptoms of diabetes insipidus. Key blood tests may include serum sodium, serum osmolality, and plasma vasopressin levels, which provide valuable information about the body's fluid balance and hormonal regulation.

In the context of diabetes insipidus, the results of blood tests can indicate whether the condition is central or nephrogenic. Central diabetes insipidus occurs when the body does not produce enough antidiuretic hormone (ADH), while nephrogenic diabetes insipidus results from the kidneys' inability to respond to this hormone. Elevated serum sodium and osmolality levels, coupled with low urine osmolality, suggest the presence of diabetes insipidus. In some cases, additional tests may be necessary to differentiate between the two types and rule out other potential causes of the symptoms.

It is also important to consider the impact of underlying conditions that may affect blood test results. For instance, patients with a history of kidney disease or those taking certain medications may exhibit altered electrolyte levels. Hormonal imbalances, particularly those related to thyroid or adrenal function, can also influence the outcomes of blood tests. Therefore, a thorough medical history and comprehensive evaluation are essential to interpret results accurately and tailor treatment accordingly.

Once a diagnosis is established, regular blood testing can be instrumental in monitoring the effectiveness of treatment and managing the condition over time. For individuals receiving medications, such as desmopressin for central diabetes insipidus, periodic blood tests help ensure that electrolyte levels remain within a safe range and that the patient is responding appropriately to therapy. These assessments play a key role in preventing potential complications associated with the condition, such as dehydration or electrolyte imbalances.

Understanding the significance of blood tests empowers patients to engage actively in their healthcare. By discussing the results with their healthcare providers, patients can gain insights into their condition and make informed decisions about their treatment options. Awareness of the implications of blood test results also highlights the importance of ongoing communication with healthcare teams, ensuring that patients receive personalized care that addresses their unique needs and concerns related to diabetes insipidus.

Imaging Studies

Imaging studies play a crucial role in the diagnosis and management of diabetes insipidus. These non-invasive techniques help healthcare providers visualize the structures within the brain and assess any underlying conditions that may contribute to the disorder. The primary imaging studies utilized include magnetic resonance imaging (MRI) and computed tomography (CT) scans. These tests are instrumental in identifying potential causes, such as tumors, cysts, or other abnormalities affecting the pituitary gland or hypothalamus, which are critical in the regulation of water balance in the body.

MRI is often the preferred method for imaging in cases of suspected diabetes insipidus. It provides detailed images of soft tissues, allowing for a comprehensive evaluation of the pituitary gland and surrounding structures. This high-resolution imaging can help detect conditions such as a pituitary adenoma or other sellar masses that may disrupt the normal function of the gland. In some cases, MRI can reveal signs of central nervous system disorders that could lead to the development of diabetes insipidus, aiding in a more accurate diagnosis.

CT scans are also valuable, particularly when MRI is contraindicated or unavailable. While CT imaging offers less detail regarding soft tissues compared to MRI, it can effectively identify larger lesions or structural abnormalities in the brain. In emergency situations, a CT scan can quickly rule out acute complications or other conditions that may mimic the symptoms of diabetes insipidus. Both imaging modalities provide essential insights that guide further diagnostic testing and treatment decisions.

In addition to MRI and CT scans, other specialized imaging techniques may be utilized based on individual patient needs. For instance, a water deprivation test or desmopressin stimulation test is essential for differentiating between central diabetes insipidus and nephrogenic diabetes insipidus. However, these tests do not involve imaging but may be conducted alongside imaging studies to provide a comprehensive assessment of the patient's condition. Understanding the results of these imaging studies is vital for patients, as it helps clarify the underlying causes of their symptoms and informs the most appropriate management strategies.

Ultimately, the findings from imaging studies can significantly impact the treatment options available for individuals with diabetes insipidus. Identifying the specific cause of the condition can lead to targeted therapies, whether it involves addressing a tumor, adjusting medications, or implementing lifestyle changes. Patients should engage in discussions with their healthcare providers about the implications of imaging results and how they fit into the overall management plan for diabetes insipidus, ensuring a collaborative approach to their healthcare journey.

Chapter 5: Treatment Options and Medications

Desmopressin

Desmopressin is a synthetic analog of vasopressin, a hormone that plays a crucial role in regulating water balance in the body. For patients living with diabetes insipidus, desmopressin serves as a fundamental treatment option. This medication is particularly effective for those with central diabetes insipidus, where the body does not produce enough vasopressin. By mimicking the action of vasopressin, desmopressin helps the kidneys concentrate urine, thereby reducing excessive urination and preventing dehydration, which are hallmark symptoms of this condition.

The administration of desmopressin can vary based on individual needs and preferences. It is available in several forms, including nasal spray, oral tablets, and subcutaneous injections. Patients may find the nasal spray particularly convenient and effective, as it provides rapid absorption and immediate relief of symptoms. Oral tablets, while also effective, may take longer to manifest their effects. The choice of administration often depends on the severity of the condition, patient lifestyle, and any potential side effects experienced with different forms.

It is important for patients to understand the dosage and frequency of desmopressin administration. Typically, the dosage is tailored to the individual, with adjustments made based on response to treatment and any side effects. Regular follow-ups with a healthcare provider are essential for monitoring response to the medication and ensuring that the treatment remains effective. Patients should be aware of the signs of both under-treatment, such as excessive thirst and urination, and over-treatment, which can lead to water retention and hyponatremia—a dangerous drop in sodium levels.

While desmopressin is generally well-tolerated, some patients may experience side effects, including headache, nausea, or nasal congestion. It is crucial for patients to discuss any side effects with their healthcare provider, who can provide guidance on managing them or adjusting the treatment regimen if necessary. Additionally, patients should be vigilant about potential interactions with other medications and inform their healthcare team of all treatments they are undergoing.

In conclusion, desmopressin plays a vital role in the management of diabetes insipidus, providing significant relief from the symptoms associated with this condition. By improving the body's ability to retain water, it enhances the quality of life for many patients. As with any medication, ongoing communication with healthcare providers about treatment efficacy and side effects is essential to optimize management strategies and ensure the best possible outcomes for individuals living with diabetes insipidus.

Thiazide Diuretics

Thiazide diuretics are a class of medications commonly used to manage various conditions, including hypertension and edema. In the context of diabetes insipidus, these medications can play a crucial role in treatment, particularly for patients with nephrogenic diabetes insipidus. Nephrogenic diabetes insipidus occurs when the kidneys fail to respond appropriately to antidiuretic hormone (ADH), leading to excessive urination and thirst. Thiazide diuretics help reduce urine output and improve the body's ability to concentrate urine, providing relief from some of the troubling symptoms associated with the condition.

The mechanism of action for thiazide diuretics is primarily related to their effect on the renal tubules. By inhibiting sodium reabsorption in the distal convoluted tubule, these medications promote sodium excretion, which leads to a decrease in urine volume. Interestingly, in patients with nephrogenic diabetes insipidus, thiazide diuretics can paradoxically decrease urine output despite their diuretic nature.

This effect is thought to arise from the enhancement of water reabsorption in the proximal tubules when sodium levels are reduced.

While thiazide diuretics can be effective, it is essential for patients to understand the potential side effects and interactions associated with their use. Common side effects may include electrolyte imbalances, such as low potassium or sodium levels, which can lead to symptoms like muscle cramps, weakness, or confusion. Regular monitoring of electrolyte levels is crucial during treatment. Additionally, it is important to discuss any other medications being taken with healthcare providers to avoid adverse interactions.

Patients should also be aware of the importance of lifestyle modifications that can complement the use of thiazide diuretics. Staying well-hydrated, consuming a balanced diet rich in potassium, and maintaining a healthy weight can enhance the effectiveness of the medication and help manage diabetes insipidus more effectively. Engaging in regular follow-up appointments with healthcare providers ensures that patients' treatment plans are adjusted as needed and that any complications are addressed promptly.

In summary, thiazide diuretics offer a valuable treatment option for individuals with nephrogenic diabetes insipidus, helping to manage symptoms and improve quality of life. Understanding their mechanism of action, potential side effects, and the role of lifestyle changes can empower patients to engage actively in their treatment. By collaborating closely with healthcare providers and monitoring their condition, patients can make informed decisions that contribute to better management of diabetes insipidus.

Managing Underlying Conditions

Managing underlying conditions that contribute to diabetes insipidus is crucial for effective treatment and overall patient well-being. Diabetes insipidus can be secondary to various medical issues, including head trauma, brain tumors, or genetic disorders affecting the production of antidiuretic hormone (ADH). Identifying and addressing these underlying conditions not only aids in managing diabetes insipidus but can also improve the patient's quality of life. Close collaboration with healthcare providers is essential to monitor these conditions and adjust treatment plans accordingly.

For patients with central diabetes insipidus, often resulting from damage to the hypothalamus or pituitary gland, it is vital to manage any neurological issues that may arise. This management may involve regular imaging studies, hormone level assessments, and possibly interventions such as surgery or radiation therapy if a tumor is involved. Additionally, medications that assist in hormone replacement or stimulate ADH production can significantly alleviate symptoms and reduce the risk of complications associated with dehydration.

In cases of nephrogenic diabetes insipidus, where the kidneys are unable to respond to ADH, managing underlying kidney conditions is key. This may include addressing chronic kidney disease, electrolyte imbalances, or side effects from certain medications. Patients should be encouraged to maintain regular appointments with their nephrologists and report any changes in kidney function or related symptoms. Dietary modifications, such as reducing sodium intake and ensuring adequate hydration, can also play a vital role in managing nephrogenic diabetes insipidus effectively.

Psychological impacts are often intertwined with the management of underlying conditions. Patients may experience anxiety or depression related to the unpredictability of their symptoms and the lifestyle adjustments required. Mental health support, including counseling or support groups, can be beneficial for coping with these challenges. Recognizing the psychological aspect of managing diabetes insipidus is pivotal for holistic treatment, ensuring that patients feel supported both physically and emotionally.

Finally, education is a powerful tool in managing underlying conditions associated with diabetes insipidus. Patients should be informed about their condition, the potential complications, and the importance of adhering to their treatment plans. Engaging in self-management strategies, such as tracking symptoms and understanding triggers, can empower patients to take an active role in their healthcare. This proactive approach fosters better communication with healthcare providers and enhances the overall management of diabetes insipidus and its underlying causes.

Monitoring and Follow-up

Monitoring and follow-up are crucial components in the management of diabetes insipidus, as they help ensure optimal health outcomes and quality of life for patients. Regular monitoring involves tracking symptoms, fluid intake, and overall hydration status. Patients should maintain a daily log of their fluid consumption, urination patterns, and any changes in symptoms. This information can provide valuable insights for healthcare providers, enabling them to make informed decisions about treatment adjustments and interventions.

Follow-up appointments with healthcare providers should be scheduled routinely to assess the effectiveness of the current treatment plan. During these visits, the healthcare team may evaluate kidney function, electrolyte levels, and the effectiveness of medications being used. It is essential for patients to communicate openly about their experiences, including any side effects they may be experiencing or any new symptoms that have emerged. This dialogue allows for timely modifications to the treatment approach, ensuring that the patient's needs are met.

Patients with diabetes insipidus may also benefit from continuous education about their condition. Understanding the signs of dehydration, recognizing when to seek medical attention, and being aware of potential complications can empower patients in their management efforts. This knowledge fosters a proactive approach, allowing individuals to take charge of their health and make informed decisions regarding their lifestyle choices and treatment adherence.

Support systems play a vital role in monitoring and follow-up as well. Family members and caregivers can assist patients by helping them keep track of their symptoms and fluid intake. They can also encourage adherence to treatment regimens and accompany patients to follow-up appointments. This collaborative approach not only enhances the effectiveness of monitoring but also provides emotional support, which is essential for coping with the challenges of living with diabetes insipidus.

Finally, utilizing technology can further enhance monitoring efforts. Mobile applications and wearable devices can track fluid intake and provide reminders for medication schedules. These tools can facilitate communication with healthcare providers by allowing patients to share real-time data about their condition. By integrating technology into their management plan, patients can achieve a more thorough understanding of their diabetes insipidus, leading to better outcomes and improved quality of life.

Chapter 6: Lifestyle Changes and Management Strategies

Hydration Strategies

Hydration strategies are crucial for managing diabetes insipidus, as the condition is characterized by excessive thirst and the excretion of large volumes of dilute urine. Patients must develop a personalized hydration plan to maintain fluid balance and prevent dehydration. This involves understanding the body's signals of thirst and recognizing the need for adequate fluid intake throughout the day. Regularly monitoring fluid intake can help patients stay mindful of their hydration status, ensuring they drink enough water to compensate for the fluid loss associated with diabetes insipidus.

One effective strategy is to establish a routine that incorporates hydration into daily activities. Setting reminders to drink water at regular intervals can help patients avoid becoming too thirsty, which often leads to excessive fluid consumption at once. Additionally, carrying a water bottle throughout the day can facilitate consistent hydration. Patients should also consider the temperature and climate, as hot weather or physical activity can increase fluid needs. It is essential to adjust fluid intake based on these factors to maintain optimal hydration levels.

Patients should also be aware of the types of liquids consumed. While water is the best option for hydration, other fluids like herbal teas or broths can also contribute to overall fluid intake. However, beverages that contain caffeine or alcohol should be limited, as they can have diuretic effects that may exacerbate fluid loss. In some cases, electrolyte-rich drinks may be beneficial, especially if a patient is losing significant amounts of fluid through urination. Consulting with a healthcare provider can help tailor these recommendations to individual needs.

In addition to liquid intake, incorporating foods with high water content into the diet can support hydration efforts. Fruits and vegetables such as cucumbers, watermelon, oranges, and strawberries can help contribute to fluid balance. These foods not only provide hydration but also essential nutrients that support overall health. Being mindful of dietary choices can enhance hydration strategies and overall well-being for individuals living with diabetes insipidus.

Finally, patients should recognize the importance of listening to their bodies and adapting hydration strategies as needed. Changes in activity level, health status, or environmental conditions can affect fluid requirements. Regular check-ins with healthcare providers can help monitor hydration status and make necessary adjustments to the hydration plan. By implementing effective hydration strategies, patients can better manage their condition and improve their quality of life.

Daily Routine Adjustments

Daily routine adjustments play a crucial role in the effective management of diabetes insipidus. Patients often experience increased thirst and urination, which can disrupt daily activities and impact overall quality of life. By making simple yet strategic changes to their routines, individuals can better accommodate their symptoms, enhance their comfort, and maintain a sense of normalcy. These adjustments can range from fluid intake schedules to planning activities around bathroom access, and they are essential for managing the condition successfully.

One of the primary adjustments involves establishing a consistent fluid intake schedule. Patients should aim to drink ample fluids throughout the day to counteract the excessive urination caused by diabetes insipidus. This may involve setting reminders to drink water at regular intervals, particularly during work or school hours when access to restrooms may be limited. Additionally, keeping a water bottle handy can serve as a visual cue to encourage hydration.

Monitoring fluid intake is also beneficial; patients may find it helpful to track their consumption to ensure they are meeting their hydration needs without overdoing it.

Incorporating regular bathroom breaks into daily activities can significantly alleviate the discomfort associated with frequent urination. Patients should plan their schedules to include ample opportunities for restroom use, particularly before long meetings, travel, or social events. Understanding one's body and recognizing the early signs of the need to urinate can help in managing these situations more effectively. Furthermore, in social settings, informing friends or colleagues about the condition can foster understanding and support, making it easier to excuse oneself when necessary.

Dietary considerations can also influence daily routines for individuals with diabetes insipidus. While there are no specific dietary restrictions for the condition, certain foods can impact fluid balance and overall health. Patients should be mindful of their salt intake, as excessive sodium can lead to increased thirst. Incorporating foods rich in water content, such as fruits and vegetables, can help maintain hydration levels. Planning meals and snacks throughout the day that align with hydration goals can contribute positively to managing symptoms and reducing the frequency of thirst.

Lastly, the psychological impact of living with diabetes insipidus should not be overlooked when making daily routine adjustments. The constant need for hydration and the potential for discomfort can lead to anxiety and stress. Establishing a routine that includes relaxation techniques, such as mindfulness or deep-breathing exercises, can help mitigate these feelings. Additionally, connecting with support groups, either in-person or online, can provide a sense of community and shared understanding among individuals facing similar challenges. By prioritizing both physical and mental well-being, patients can navigate their daily lives with greater ease and confidence.

Exercise Considerations

Exercise considerations for individuals with diabetes insipidus (DI) are essential to ensure that physical activity contributes positively to overall health and well-being. While exercise offers numerous benefits, such as improved cardiovascular health, weight management, and enhanced mood, patients with DI must approach their fitness routines with caution. The primary concern for individuals with this condition is the potential for dehydration, given that DI is characterized by an inability to concentrate urine, leading to excessive fluid loss. Therefore, it is vital to stay well-hydrated before, during, and after exercise to mitigate the risk of dehydration.

Before starting any exercise program, patients should consult with their healthcare provider to determine the appropriate type and intensity of exercise. Each individual's situation is unique, and factors such as the underlying cause of DI, overall health status, and fitness level must be considered. Low-impact exercises, such as walking, swimming, or cycling, can be particularly beneficial, as they are less likely to exacerbate symptoms. It is also advisable to incorporate flexibility and strength training exercises to enhance overall fitness and support joint health.

Hydration strategies should be a key component of any exercise plan for individuals with DI. Patients should aim to drink fluids regularly throughout the day, with a focus on water and electrolyte-rich beverages. It is recommended to carry a water bottle during workouts and to schedule breaks to rehydrate, especially during prolonged or intense physical activities. Monitoring urine output and color can serve as a practical guide; patients should strive for a light yellow color, which indicates proper hydration.

Additionally, it is important to be aware of the signs of dehydration and to take them seriously. Symptoms such as dizziness, dry mouth, fatigue, and increased thirst may indicate that hydration levels are becoming inadequate. If any of these signs occur during exercise, it is crucial to stop, rest, and hydrate immediately. Patients should also consider adjusting their exercise schedule to avoid extreme temperatures, as heat and humidity can significantly increase fluid loss.

Finally, incorporating exercise into daily routines can provide psychological benefits, fostering a sense of control and well-being amidst the challenges of managing diabetes insipidus. Group activities or classes can also offer social support, which is valuable for emotional health. By focusing on appropriate exercise considerations, individuals with DI can enjoy the benefits of physical activity while effectively managing their condition.

Stress Management Techniques

Stress can significantly impact the management of diabetes insipidus, making stress management techniques essential for patients navigating this condition. Stress often exacerbates symptoms and can lead to complications, so implementing effective strategies is crucial. Techniques such as deep breathing exercises, progressive muscle relaxation, and mindfulness meditation can help reduce stress levels. These methods promote relaxation and can help patients regain a sense of control over their symptoms, ultimately improving their overall well-being.

Another effective approach is physical activity, which has been shown to reduce stress and improve mood. Regular exercise can also help maintain a healthy weight and promote better hydration, both of which are important for managing diabetes insipidus. Activities like walking, swimming, or yoga can be tailored to individual preferences and physical abilities, making it easier for patients to incorporate them into their daily routines. Establishing a consistent exercise schedule can provide additional structure and predictability, which may further alleviate stress.

Social support plays a vital role in stress management as well. Connecting with friends, family, or support groups can provide an emotional outlet and valuable resources for coping with the challenges of diabetes insipidus. Sharing experiences and strategies with others who understand the condition can foster a sense of community and belonging. Patients should consider participating in local or online support groups to discuss their feelings and exchange information, which can enhance their emotional resilience.

Time management and organization are also critical components of stress management. Patients can benefit from creating a structured daily routine that includes time for self-care, medication management, and hydration. Utilizing tools such as planners, reminders, or mobile applications can help keep track of necessary tasks and reduce feelings of overwhelm. By prioritizing and breaking down responsibilities into manageable steps, patients can cultivate a sense of accomplishment and reduce the stress associated with feeling unprepared.

Lastly, seeking professional help when needed is crucial for managing stress effectively. Mental health professionals can provide support through counseling or therapy, helping patients develop coping strategies tailored to their specific situations. Cognitive-behavioral techniques, for instance, can aid individuals in changing negative thought patterns that contribute to stress. By addressing both the psychological and practical aspects of stress management, patients can enhance their quality of life while living with diabetes insipidus.

Chapter 7: Diabetes Insipidus in Children

Symptoms in Pediatric Patients

Diabetes insipidus (DI) in pediatric patients often presents with distinct symptoms that can significantly impact a child's daily life and well-being. One of the most common indicators of DI in children is excessive thirst, known as polydipsia. Children may frequently request water and demonstrate an insatiable thirst that can lead to increased fluid intake. This symptom can be particularly challenging for parents and caregivers, as it may be mistaken for typical childhood behavior or a result of hot weather or physical activity. It is essential to differentiate between normal thirst and the persistent craving for fluids that characterizes DI.

Another hallmark symptom of diabetes insipidus is polyuria, which refers to the production of large volumes of urine. In children, this can manifest as frequent urination, often leading to bedwetting in those who are previously toilet trained. Parents may notice that their child requires frequent changes of clothing and bedding due to this symptom. The increased urination can also lead to dehydration, which may result in additional symptoms such as dry skin, fatigue, and irritability. Parents should be vigilant in monitoring their child's urinary habits to identify potential signs of DI.

In addition to excessive thirst and urination, children with diabetes insipidus may experience weight loss or failure to thrive, especially in young children and infants. The loss of fluids can hinder proper growth and development, prompting concerns about nutritional intake and overall health. Parents should be aware that if a child is not gaining weight as expected or appears to be losing weight, it could indicate an underlying issue such as DI. Early recognition of these signs is crucial for timely intervention and management.

Behavioral changes can also be an important symptom of diabetes insipidus in pediatric patients. Children may exhibit increased irritability, mood swings, or lethargy, particularly when they are dehydrated. These behavioral changes can often be attributed to discomfort or the physical effects of dehydration, making it essential for caregivers to consider the possibility of DI if such symptoms persist. Monitoring a child's emotional and physical state can provide valuable insights into their overall health and help identify the need for medical evaluation.

Finally, it is crucial for parents and caregivers to communicate any concerns regarding their child's symptoms to healthcare professionals. Diagnosis and management of diabetes insipidus in children require a collaborative approach involving physicians, caregivers, and sometimes specialists. By recognizing the symptoms of DI early and seeking appropriate medical advice, families can ensure their child receives the necessary care and support, leading to improved quality of life and better outcomes.

Diagnosis and Testing in Children

Diagnosis of diabetes insipidus in children begins with a thorough evaluation of symptoms and medical history. Parents often notice excessive thirst and frequent urination in their children, which may prompt them to seek medical advice. It is essential for healthcare providers to differentiate between the two main types of diabetes insipidus: central diabetes insipidus, which results from a deficiency of the hormone vasopressin, and nephrogenic diabetes insipidus, where the kidneys are unable to respond to this hormone. The child's age, growth patterns, and overall health can also influence the diagnostic process.

The first step in testing for diabetes insipidus typically involves a physical exam and a detailed review of the child's symptoms. Physicians may also conduct urinalysis to measure the concentration of urine. In children with diabetes insipidus, urine is usually very dilute, indicating that the kidneys are not properly concentrating urine. Blood tests can also help assess the levels of electrolytes and hormones, providing insight into kidney function and the body's ability to regulate water balance.

A water deprivation test is often employed to confirm the diagnosis. During this test, the child is monitored in a controlled environment where fluid intake is restricted. This helps determine how the body responds to dehydration and whether vasopressin levels are adequate. If the child continues to produce large amounts of dilute urine despite the lack of fluid intake, it may suggest nephrogenic diabetes insipidus. Conversely, if urine concentration improves after administration of vasopressin, it indicates central diabetes insipidus.

Imaging studies, such as MRI scans, may also be utilized to examine the pituitary gland and hypothalamus, which are crucial in the production of vasopressin. Identifying any structural abnormalities in these areas can aid in determining the cause of diabetes insipidus. Genetic testing may be warranted in certain cases, especially if there is a family history of the condition or if symptoms appear at a very young age.

Accurate diagnosis and testing are vital for effective management of diabetes insipidus in children. Early identification allows for timely intervention, which can significantly improve the quality of life for affected children. Once diagnosed, healthcare providers can develop an appropriate treatment plan tailored to the child's specific needs, ensuring both medical and emotional support for the child and their family.

Treatment Approaches for Children

Treatment approaches for children diagnosed with diabetes insipidus vary significantly from those designed for adults, primarily due to the unique physiological and emotional needs of younger patients. The first step in treatment typically involves determining the underlying cause of the condition, which can be either central diabetes insipidus or nephrogenic diabetes insipidus. While central diabetes insipidus is often caused by damage to the hypothalamus or pituitary gland, nephrogenic diabetes insipidus usually results from a genetic mutation or acquired factors affecting the kidneys. A careful assessment by a pediatric endocrinologist is essential for establishing an accurate diagnosis and tailoring an appropriate treatment plan.

For children with central diabetes insipidus, desmopressin, a synthetic form of the antidiuretic hormone vasopressin, is commonly prescribed. This medication helps the kidneys concentrate urine, thereby reducing excessive urination and thirst. Desmopressin can be administered as a nasal spray or in oral form, and its dosage is adjusted based on the child's age, weight, and response to treatment. Regular monitoring is crucial to ensure that the child receives the correct dose, as both under-treatment and over-treatment can lead to complications. For nephrogenic diabetes insipidus, treatment may involve the use of diuretics in conjunction with dietary modifications to manage symptoms effectively.

In addition to pharmacological interventions, lifestyle modifications play a vital role in managing diabetes insipidus in children. Parents and caregivers should encourage regular fluid intake, ensuring that the child remains well-hydrated throughout the day. Offering a variety of fluids can help maintain interest and compliance. It may also be beneficial to establish a routine for bathroom breaks, especially during school hours, to minimize accidents and discomfort. Education about the condition is essential, not only for the child but also for teachers and caregivers, to foster an understanding of the child's needs and to ensure a supportive environment.

Psychological support is another critical component of treatment for children with diabetes insipidus. The condition can affect a child's emotional well-being and social interactions, leading to anxiety or feelings of isolation. Engaging with a mental health professional who specializes in pediatric care may help address these emotional concerns. Support groups for children can also provide a safe space for sharing experiences and coping strategies. Encouraging open communication about feelings and challenges related to diabetes insipidus can empower children to advocate for their needs and foster resilience.

Finally, ongoing follow-up appointments are essential for monitoring the child's growth, development, and response to treatment. Regular check-ups allow healthcare providers to make necessary adjustments to the treatment plan and ensure that the child is thriving. As children grow, their needs may change, requiring modifications to their medication or management strategies. Collaborating closely with a healthcare team composed of pediatricians, endocrinologists, dietitians, and mental health professionals will provide a comprehensive approach to treatment, ultimately leading to improved health outcomes and quality of life for children living with diabetes insipidus.

Support for Families

Support for families dealing with diabetes insipidus is crucial, as the condition not only affects the individual diagnosed but also has a significant impact on family dynamics. Understanding the nature of diabetes insipidus and its implications can help families navigate the challenges that arise. Families must be aware of the symptoms, treatment options, and management strategies to provide the necessary support to their loved ones. This knowledge empowers them to create a nurturing environment that fosters both understanding and compassion.

Education plays a key role in supporting families. By learning about the causes and risk factors of diabetes insipidus, family members can better comprehend the condition and its effects. This understanding can alleviate fears and misconceptions that may arise. Families should take advantage of resources such as support groups, educational workshops, and reputable online materials to gain insights into the daily realities of living with diabetes insipidus. Being informed allows family members to advocate more effectively for their loved ones and engage with healthcare providers in meaningful discussions.

Open communication within the family is essential for managing diabetes insipidus effectively. Encouraging discussions about symptoms, treatment options, and emotional challenges can help foster a supportive atmosphere. Families should create a space where individuals feel comfortable sharing their experiences and concerns. This dialogue can lead to better coping strategies for all involved, as well as help identify specific needs that may arise. By working together, families can develop practical solutions to everyday challenges, such as managing fluid intake and recognizing when to seek medical attention.

The psychological impact of diabetes insipidus can be significant, and families must be prepared to address emotional and mental health needs. Individuals may experience feelings of isolation, frustration, or anxiety related to their condition. Family members should be attentive to these emotional changes and encourage open discussions about feelings and coping mechanisms. Seeking professional counseling or support groups can also provide valuable resources for both patients and their families. By acknowledging and addressing these psychological aspects, families can help their loved ones feel less alone in their journey.

Lastly, practical support can make a substantial difference in the daily lives of families affected by diabetes insipidus. This may include helping with medication management, maintaining a hydration schedule, or assisting with dietary considerations. Family members can also play a role in encouraging healthy lifestyle changes that contribute to better management of the condition. By actively participating in the care process, families reinforce their support and commitment, fostering a sense of unity and resilience. Through education, communication, emotional support, and practical assistance, families can create an environment that promotes better health and well-being for their loved ones with diabetes insipidus.

Chapter 8: Psychological Impact of Living with Diabetes Insipidus

Emotional Challenges

Emotional challenges associated with diabetes insipidus can be profound and multifaceted, affecting both patients and their caregivers. Living with a chronic condition often brings about feelings of uncertainty, anxiety, and frustration. Patients may struggle with the constant need to manage their hydration levels, which can lead to a sense of loss of control over their daily lives. The burden of frequent bathroom trips and the need to carry water at all times can also contribute to social anxiety, making it difficult for individuals to engage in normal activities or attend social events.

The psychological impact of diabetes insipidus can lead to increased stress and emotional strain. Patients may experience feelings of isolation, especially if they perceive that others do not understand their condition or its implications. This emotional toll can be compounded by the need for ongoing medical appointments and potential lifestyle adjustments. It is not uncommon for patients to feel overwhelmed by the prospect of managing a chronic illness, leading to depression or anxiety disorders that can further affect their quality of life.

Caregivers also face emotional challenges as they support their loved ones with diabetes insipidus. They may experience feelings of helplessness when they witness the struggles of the patient and may grapple with their own worries about the future. The dynamics of caregiving can lead to stress, burnout, and even resentment if the caregiver feels their own needs are being neglected. Open communication between patients and caregivers is crucial to navigate these emotional difficulties and provide mutual support.

Coping strategies play a vital role in addressing the emotional challenges of diabetes insipidus. Encouraging patients to join support groups can foster a sense of community and understanding, allowing them to share their experiences and learn from others who are facing similar challenges. Additionally, engaging in mindfulness practices, such as meditation or yoga, can help reduce stress and improve emotional well-being. It is essential for both patients and caregivers to prioritize self-care and seek professional help if feelings of anxiety or depression become overwhelming.

Overall, recognizing and addressing the emotional challenges associated with diabetes insipidus is critical for improving the overall quality of life for patients and their families. By fostering open communication, utilizing coping strategies, and seeking support when needed, individuals can better manage the psychological impacts of the condition. This holistic approach not only enhances emotional resilience but also contributes to a more positive outlook on living with diabetes insipidus.

Support Systems

Support systems play a crucial role in managing diabetes insipidus, providing patients with the resources, emotional backing, and practical assistance needed to navigate their condition. A well-structured support system can help individuals cope with the complexities of diabetes insipidus, which may include frequent urination, excessive thirst, and the potential complications that arise from these symptoms. Understanding the various elements of a support system can empower patients to take an active role in their health management and foster resilience in the face of challenges.

Family and friends are often the first line of support for individuals diagnosed with diabetes insipidus. Their understanding, patience, and encouragement can significantly impact a patient's emotional well-being. It is important for patients to communicate openly with their loved ones about their condition, sharing specific needs and concerns. This dialogue not only helps family and friends understand the challenges faced by the patient but also fosters a supportive environment where patients feel safe discussing their experiences and seeking help when necessary.

Healthcare professionals, including endocrinologists, nurses, and dietitians, form another vital component of the support system. These professionals can provide comprehensive information about the condition, its causes, and the latest treatment options available. Regular check-ups and consultations with healthcare experts are essential for monitoring the disease and adjusting treatment plans as needed. Patients should feel comfortable asking questions and expressing any concerns during these appointments, as this engagement can lead to better health outcomes and a more tailored approach to management.

Support groups, whether in-person or online, offer an additional layer of assistance for those living with diabetes insipidus. Connecting with others who share similar experiences can alleviate feelings of isolation and provide valuable insights into coping strategies. Support groups often facilitate discussions on practical management techniques, such as lifestyle modifications and dietary considerations. Patients can share tips, resources, and emotional support, creating a sense of community that is beneficial for mental health.

Lastly, psychological support is an essential aspect of a comprehensive support system for individuals with diabetes insipidus. Living with a chronic condition can lead to stress, anxiety, and feelings of frustration. Professional counseling or therapy can help patients process these emotions, develop coping strategies, and enhance their overall quality of life. Recognizing the importance of mental health in chronic illness management underscores the need for a holistic approach, where emotional and psychological well-being is prioritized alongside physical health.

Coping Mechanisms

Coping mechanisms are essential for individuals living with diabetes insipidus as they navigate the challenges associated with this condition. Understanding the emotional and psychological landscape can empower patients to manage their symptoms more effectively. Recognizing that diabetes insipidus may lead to feelings of frustration, anxiety, or isolation is the first step in developing robust coping strategies. Patients often benefit from identifying their emotions and acknowledging that they are not alone in their experiences. Support systems, whether through family, friends, or support groups, can provide a crucial buffer against these feelings.

One effective coping mechanism is education. Gaining a comprehensive understanding of diabetes insipidus, including its causes, symptoms, and treatment options, helps patients feel more in control of their condition. Knowledge can alleviate fears and uncertainties, making it easier to engage with healthcare providers and advocate for appropriate care. Patients are encouraged to ask questions, seek information from reputable sources, and participate in educational workshops or support groups. This proactive approach fosters a sense of empowerment and can significantly improve overall well-being.

Another vital aspect of coping involves the establishment of a daily routine that accommodates the unique challenges posed by diabetes insipidus. Implementing strategies such as setting reminders for medication, maintaining a consistent fluid intake schedule, and tracking symptoms can help individuals manage their condition more effectively. Additionally, incorporating stress-reducing activities like mindfulness, yoga, or gentle exercise can enhance emotional resilience. Patients should also consider maintaining a balanced diet to support overall health, which can further mitigate some of the stressors associated with managing diabetes insipidus.

Emotional support is crucial for coping with the psychological impact of living with diabetes insipidus. Engaging with mental health professionals can provide patients with tools to manage anxiety and depression that may arise from the condition. Cognitive-behavioral therapy, for instance, can assist individuals in reframing negative thoughts and developing healthier coping strategies. Peer support groups, whether in-person or online, offer a platform for sharing experiences and strategies, reducing feelings of isolation. Building connections with others who understand the daily realities of diabetes insipidus can foster a sense of community.

Lastly, caregivers also play a significant role in the coping mechanisms of patients with diabetes insipidus. They should be educated about the condition and its effects to provide effective support. Caregivers may need to establish their own coping strategies to manage the emotional toll of caregiving. Encouraging open communication between patients and caregivers can strengthen relationships and improve the quality of care. By working together, both patients and caregivers can create a supportive environment that fosters resilience and promotes better management of diabetes insipidus.

Seeking Professional Help

Seeking professional help is a crucial step for anyone experiencing symptoms related to diabetes insipidus. The condition, characterized by excessive thirst and urination, can significantly impact daily life and overall well-being. Understanding when and why to consult a healthcare provider can empower patients to take control of their health. Early diagnosis and intervention are essential, as untreated diabetes insipidus can lead to complications that affect both physical and psychological health.

When approaching a healthcare professional, patients should be prepared to discuss their symptoms in detail. It is important to note the frequency and volume of urination, the level of thirst, and any other related symptoms. This information helps healthcare providers assess the condition accurately. Additionally, patients should inform their doctors about their medical history, including any medications they are taking, which may influence the diagnosis. Comprehensive information enables providers to rule out other potential causes and focus on an accurate diagnosis of diabetes insipidus.

Diagnosis of diabetes insipidus typically involves a series of tests. These may include a water deprivation test, which assesses the body's ability to concentrate urine under controlled conditions. Blood tests may also be conducted to measure levels of hormones such as vasopressin, which regulates water retention. Understanding the diagnostic process can help patients feel more at ease and prepared for what to expect during their medical appointments. Being informed can reduce anxiety and foster a collaborative relationship with healthcare providers.

Once diagnosed, patients will need to explore treatment options. The approach may vary depending on the type of diabetes insipidus, whether central or nephrogenic. Treatment may involve medications that help manage symptoms, such as desmopressin for central diabetes insipidus. Along with pharmacological interventions, lifestyle changes can play a significant role in managing the condition. Patients should discuss with their healthcare providers about dietary considerations and hydration strategies that can help alleviate symptoms and enhance quality of life.

Lastly, it is crucial for patients to recognize the psychological impact of living with diabetes insipidus. The constant need to drink water and frequent urination can lead to feelings of isolation, frustration, or anxiety. Seeking support from mental health professionals or joining support groups can be beneficial. Patients are encouraged to communicate their emotional needs with their healthcare providers, who can offer resources or referrals to help manage the psychological aspects of living with diabetes insipidus. Understanding that seeking professional help encompasses both physical and emotional health is vital for holistic management of the condition.

Chapter 9: Dietary Considerations

Nutritional Needs

Nutritional needs for individuals with diabetes insipidus focus on maintaining overall health while managing the condition's unique challenges. Since diabetes insipidus results in the frequent excretion of large volumes of diluted urine, hydration becomes a critical aspect of dietary management. Patients should prioritize fluid intake, ensuring they consume adequate amounts of water throughout the day. In some cases, electrolyte-rich beverages may also be beneficial, as they can help restore balance and prevent dehydration. Consulting with a healthcare provider or dietitian can provide personalized recommendations based on individual health status and activity levels.

In addition to hydration, a well-balanced diet plays a significant role in managing diabetes insipidus. Incorporating a variety of fruits, vegetables, whole grains, lean proteins, and healthy fats can support overall well-being. Patients should focus on nutrient-dense foods that provide essential vitamins and minerals, as these contribute to optimal bodily functions. Particular attention should be given to foods rich in potassium and magnesium, as these nutrients can help maintain proper fluid balance and support kidney function.

Monitoring sodium intake is also crucial for individuals with diabetes insipidus, especially those with nephrogenic diabetes insipidus, where the kidneys are less responsive to antidiuretic hormone. High sodium levels can exacerbate thirst and increase urine output, making it harder to maintain proper hydration. A diet low in processed foods, which often contain high levels of sodium, can help mitigate these effects. Patients should read food labels carefully and opt for fresh, whole foods whenever possible.

Moreover, the psychological impact of living with diabetes insipidus may influence eating habits and nutritional choices. Anxiety and stress can lead to poor dietary decisions, which could negatively affect overall health. It is essential for patients to adopt mindful eating practices, taking the time to plan meals and snacks that align with their nutritional needs. Engaging in support groups or therapy can also provide valuable coping strategies, helping patients navigate the emotional aspects of their condition while fostering healthier eating behaviors.

Finally, patients should remain proactive in discussing their nutritional needs with their healthcare team. Regular check-ins can help track any changes in health status, and adjustments to dietary recommendations may be necessary over time. By understanding and addressing their nutritional needs, individuals with diabetes insipidus can better manage their condition, enhance their quality of life, and reduce the risk of potential complications associated with the disorder.

Hydration and Diet

Hydration plays a crucial role in the management of diabetes insipidus, a condition characterized by the excretion of large volumes of dilute urine due to inadequate action of the hormone vasopressin. Patients must prioritize maintaining proper fluid intake to prevent dehydration, which can lead to a range of complications. It is essential to drink fluids regularly throughout the day, especially if you are experiencing excessive thirst or have increased urination. Understanding your body's hydration needs is vital, and keeping a close eye on fluid intake can help manage symptoms effectively.

Diet also plays an integral part in managing diabetes insipidus. While there are no specific dietary restrictions, a balanced diet rich in fruits, vegetables, whole grains, and lean proteins can support overall health and well-being. Certain foods may have a higher water content, such as cucumbers, watermelon, and oranges, which can contribute to hydration. Monitoring your diet can help you identify which foods make you feel your best and support your fluid balance. Additionally, incorporating sources of electrolytes, such as potassium and sodium, can help maintain proper bodily functions, especially when fluid loss is significant.

While the primary focus for individuals with diabetes insipidus is hydration, attention should also be given to the timing of fluid intake. Spreading fluid consumption throughout the day rather than consuming large amounts at once can prevent abrupt changes in hydration levels. It is important to consider your daily activities; for instance, if you are exercising or spending time in a hot environment, you may need to increase your fluid intake to compensate for potential losses through sweat. Keeping a water bottle handy and setting reminders to drink can help create a routine that supports adequate hydration.

In some cases, dietary modifications may also play a role in addressing specific symptoms related to diabetes insipidus. For instance, reducing caffeine and alcohol intake can help minimize their diuretic effects, allowing for better hydration. Additionally, a diet low in added sugars and refined carbohydrates can aid in overall health, as these foods may contribute to fluctuations in energy levels and affect your body's ability to maintain balance. Consulting with a registered dietitian or healthcare provider can provide personalized dietary recommendations tailored to your needs.

Lastly, it is important to recognize the psychological aspects of managing hydration and diet in diabetes insipidus. The constant need to monitor fluid intake and the potential for dietary limitations can create stress and anxiety for some individuals. Engaging in mindful eating practices and finding supportive communities can help alleviate some of these pressures. Building a routine that includes healthy hydration and eating habits can empower patients to take control of their condition, leading to improved quality of life and better management of diabetes insipidus.

Foods to Include and Avoid

Dietary choices play a significant role in managing diabetes insipidus, a condition characterized by excessive thirst and urination due to the body's inability to regulate water balance. While there is no specific diet for diabetes insipidus, certain foods can help alleviate symptoms and maintain overall health. Patients should focus on including hydrating foods in their diet, such as fruits and vegetables with high water content. Examples include cucumbers, watermelon, oranges, and strawberries. These foods not only provide hydration but also essential vitamins and minerals that support overall bodily functions.

In addition to hydrating foods, incorporating whole grains, lean proteins, and healthy fats can contribute to better health outcomes. Whole grains such as brown rice, quinoa, and oats provide necessary fiber, which can help regulate blood sugar levels and improve digestive health. Lean proteins, including chicken, fish, and legumes, are essential for maintaining muscle mass and promoting satiety. Healthy fats from sources like avocados, nuts, and olive oil can also support cardiovascular health, which is crucial for patients managing any chronic condition.

Conversely, certain foods should be minimized or avoided to help manage diabetes insipidus symptoms effectively. High-sodium foods, such as processed snacks, canned soups, and fast food, can lead to increased thirst and exacerbate fluid imbalance. Patients should be mindful of their salt intake and choose fresh, unprocessed foods whenever possible. Sugary drinks and beverages, including soda and fruit juices, should also be limited as they can contribute to dehydration and lead to fluctuations in blood sugar levels, further complicating overall health management.

Caffeine and alcohol are two other categories of foods and beverages that individuals with diabetes insipidus should approach with caution. Caffeine can act as a diuretic, potentially increasing urine output and leading to further dehydration. Alcohol can also have a dehydrating effect and may interfere with medication effectiveness. Patients should discuss their consumption of these substances with their healthcare provider to determine the best approach for their specific situation.

Overall, adopting a balanced and mindful approach to eating can significantly impact the management of diabetes insipidus. By including hydrating foods and avoiding those that can exacerbate symptoms, patients can work towards better hydration and overall health. It is essential to consult with a healthcare professional or a registered dietitian for personalized dietary advice tailored to individual needs and circumstances. This can help ensure that dietary choices support not only the management of diabetes insipidus but also overall well-being.

Meal Planning Tips

Meal planning is an essential strategy for managing diabetes insipidus effectively. By organizing meals ahead of time, patients can better control their fluid intake, ensure a balanced diet, and mitigate potential complications associated with the condition. The key is to create a meal plan that accommodates both dietary needs and personal preferences while being mindful of hydration levels. A well-structured meal plan not only alleviates the stress of last-minute decisions but also promotes healthier eating habits, which can lead to improved overall well-being.

When planning meals, consider incorporating a variety of foods from all food groups to ensure a balanced intake of nutrients. Focus on fruits, vegetables, whole grains, lean proteins, and healthy fats. These components are vital for maintaining energy levels and supporting overall health. Additionally, patients should be aware of their individual dietary restrictions, particularly if they are on medications that may require monitoring of sodium or potassium intake. Working with a registered dietitian familiar with diabetes insipidus can provide personalized guidance tailored to specific health needs.

Hydration is a crucial aspect of meal planning for individuals with diabetes insipidus. Since the condition often leads to excessive urination and thirst, it is important to develop strategies that ensure adequate fluid intake throughout the day. Incorporating hydrating foods such as cucumbers, watermelon, and soups can help increase overall fluid consumption. It's helpful to set reminders to drink water at regular intervals and to keep a water bottle accessible to promote consistent hydration. Balancing fluid intake with meals can also help manage thirst levels.

Portion control plays a significant role in meal planning and can help prevent overeating. Using smaller plates or measuring portions can assist in managing caloric intake while ensuring a balanced diet. It is beneficial to pre-portion snacks and meals to reduce the temptation of consuming excessive amounts, particularly when managing cravings. Additionally, patients should be mindful of the timing of their meals, as regular meal intervals can help regulate hunger and thirst signals, further supporting fluid management.

Finally, flexibility is key in meal planning for individuals with diabetes insipidus. While it is important to have a plan, being adaptable allows for changes in daily routines or unexpected circumstances. This can include substituting ingredients based on availability or adjusting meal times based on hunger cues. Keeping a food journal can also be a useful tool to track food intake, hydration levels, and how these factors correlate with overall health. By embracing a flexible yet structured approach to meal planning, patients can better manage their condition and improve their quality of life.

Chapter 10: Complications and Long-term Effects

Potential Complications

Potential complications of diabetes insipidus can arise due to the underlying causes of the condition as well as the effects of living with it. One of the most significant complications is dehydration, which can occur if the individual is unable to maintain adequate fluid intake to compensate for excessive urination. Chronic dehydration can lead to serious health issues, including kidney damage, electrolyte imbalances, and decreased overall organ function. Understanding the signs of dehydration, such as dry mouth, increased thirst, and dizziness, is crucial for patients to manage their condition effectively.

Another potential complication involves the psychological impact of diabetes insipidus. Living with a chronic condition can lead to anxiety, depression, and feelings of isolation. Patients may feel overwhelmed by the constant need to monitor fluid intake and output, which can disrupt their daily lives. Support networks, counseling, and educational resources can play a vital role in helping patients cope with these emotional challenges, as addressing mental health is as important as managing physical symptoms.

Furthermore, diabetes insipidus can affect the management of other health conditions. For patients with concurrent illnesses such as diabetes mellitus or cardiovascular diseases, the interplay of these conditions can complicate treatment plans. Medications for diabetes or blood pressure may interact with treatments for diabetes insipidus, necessitating careful monitoring and adjustments by healthcare providers. Patients should communicate openly with their medical team about all medications and conditions to ensure a coordinated approach to their health.

Long-term effects of untreated or poorly managed diabetes insipidus can lead to chronic kidney disease. The kidneys are responsible for filtering excess fluids, and when they are consistently overworked due to excessive urination, they can become damaged over time. Regular check-ups and kidney function tests are essential for patients to monitor their renal health and prevent complications that could arise from prolonged fluid imbalance.

Lastly, lifestyle changes can significantly impact the risk of complications associated with diabetes insipidus. Implementing strategies such as maintaining a balanced diet, staying hydrated, and adhering to prescribed treatment plans can enhance overall health and quality of life. Patients are encouraged to engage in regular physical activity, manage stress effectively, and seek education on their condition to better navigate the challenges they face. By taking proactive steps, individuals with diabetes insipidus can reduce the likelihood of complications and lead fulfilling lives.

Long-term Health Considerations

Long-term health considerations for individuals with diabetes insipidus are crucial for maintaining overall well-being and preventing potential complications. One of the primary concerns is the risk of dehydration, which can occur if the body's ability to concentrate urine is impaired. Patients must remain vigilant about their fluid intake to ensure they are adequately hydrated. Chronic dehydration can lead to various health issues, including kidney damage, urinary tract infections, and other complications that may further complicate the management of diabetes insipidus.

Another significant consideration is the impact of diabetes insipidus on electrolyte balance. Since this condition often leads to excessive urination, it can result in imbalances in sodium and potassium levels. Monitoring these electrolyte levels regularly is essential, as fluctuations can affect heart function and lead to other systemic health issues. Patients should work closely with their healthcare providers to establish a routine for monitoring and adjusting dietary intake or medications as needed.

Long-term management of diabetes insipidus also requires awareness of potential psychological effects. Living with a chronic condition can lead to anxiety, depression, and social isolation. Patients may feel burdened by the constant need to manage their fluid intake and urination schedule, which can affect their quality of life. Support from healthcare professionals, support groups, and mental health resources can provide valuable assistance in coping with these emotional challenges.

In addition to psychological considerations, lifestyle modifications play a vital role in managing diabetes insipidus. Patients are encouraged to adopt a balanced diet, maintain a regular exercise regimen, and establish consistent daily routines. These adjustments can help regulate fluid intake and improve overall health. It is also important for patients to educate themselves about their condition, enabling them to make informed decisions regarding their treatment and lifestyle choices.

Finally, regular follow-up appointments with healthcare providers are essential for monitoring the long-term effects of diabetes insipidus. These visits allow for the assessment of kidney function, electrolyte levels, and the effectiveness of current treatment strategies. Staying proactive about health management can help minimize complications and promote a better quality of life for individuals living with diabetes insipidus. By understanding the long-term implications of their condition, patients can take an active role in their health and well-being.

Monitoring for Complications

Monitoring for complications in diabetes insipidus is a crucial aspect of managing the condition effectively. Patients should be aware of the potential complications that can arise and the importance of regular monitoring to prevent them. Diabetes insipidus can lead to significant fluid imbalances, which may result in dehydration or electrolyte disturbances. Therefore, understanding how to monitor these risks is essential for maintaining overall health and well-being.

Regular check-ups with healthcare providers are vital for individuals with diabetes insipidus. These appointments often include monitoring fluid intake and output, as well as assessing weight changes. Patients should keep a daily log of their fluid consumption and any symptoms they experience. This information can help healthcare professionals identify patterns and make necessary adjustments to treatment plans. In addition, periodic blood tests may be conducted to evaluate electrolyte levels, kidney function, and overall metabolic status.

Another important aspect of monitoring for complications is recognizing the signs and symptoms of dehydration. Patients should be educated about the early indicators of dehydration, such as increased thirst, dry mouth, fatigue, and dizziness. Prompt recognition of these signs can lead to quicker interventions, such as increasing fluid intake or adjusting medications. Furthermore, understanding the risks associated with dehydration, including the potential for kidney damage, can empower patients to take proactive measures in their daily lives.

Patients should also be aware of the psychological impact of living with diabetes insipidus, which can indirectly contribute to complications. Anxiety and stress can exacerbate symptoms, leading to fluctuations in fluid balance. Therefore, it is essential to incorporate mental health monitoring into the overall management plan. Support groups or counseling may provide valuable resources for coping with the emotional challenges of the condition, ensuring that patients maintain a holistic approach to their health.

Finally, education on dietary considerations is important for preventing complications related to diabetes insipidus. A balanced diet that supports hydration and electrolyte balance can play a significant role in management. Patients should consult with nutritionists to develop meal plans that consider their condition and lifestyle. By being proactive in monitoring their health and understanding the potential complications associated with diabetes insipidus, patients can significantly improve their quality of life and reduce the risk of serious health issues.

Importance of Regular Check-ups

Regular check-ups are a crucial component of managing diabetes insipidus effectively. These appointments provide an opportunity for patients to monitor their condition, assess the effectiveness of treatment, and make necessary adjustments. By maintaining a routine schedule of visits to healthcare providers, individuals with diabetes insipidus can ensure that they receive timely evaluations and interventions, which can significantly improve their quality of life. Regular check-ups help identify any emerging complications early, allowing for prompt management and reducing the risk of severe health issues.

During these visits, healthcare professionals conduct thorough assessments that may include reviewing symptoms, conducting laboratory tests, and evaluating hydration levels. This comprehensive approach helps in understanding how well the body is responding to treatment and whether any changes in medication or lifestyle are needed. For instance, fluctuations in urine output or thirst levels can provide vital clues about the effectiveness of antidiuretic hormone replacement therapies or other treatment options. Patients are encouraged to communicate openly about their experiences, as this information is vital for tailoring their management plan.

In addition to monitoring physical health, regular check-ups also address the psychological aspects of living with diabetes insipidus. Many patients experience anxiety or emotional distress related to their condition, and healthcare providers can offer support and resources to help manage these feelings. Mental health screenings during check-ups can identify issues that may need further attention, enabling patients to receive holistic care that addresses both their physical and emotional needs. Understanding that diabetes insipidus can have psychological impacts encourages open discussions about mental well-being, which is essential for comprehensive care.

Moreover, regular check-ups serve as an educational platform for patients. Healthcare providers can offer updated information about diabetes insipidus, including new treatment options, dietary recommendations, and lifestyle changes that can enhance management. Patients can learn about the importance of hydration, the role of diet in managing symptoms, and strategies for coping with the condition in daily life. This ongoing education empowers patients to take an active role in their health, fostering a sense of control and encouraging adherence to recommended management strategies.

Finally, the importance of building a strong patient-provider relationship cannot be overstated. Regular check-ups allow patients to establish trust and rapport with their healthcare team, which is vital for effective communication and individualized care. Patients who feel comfortable discussing their concerns and experiences are more likely to adhere to treatment plans and take proactive steps in their health management. As such, regular check-ups not only facilitate physical health monitoring but also enhance the overall patient experience, ultimately contributing to better health outcomes in individuals living with diabetes insipidus.

Chapter 11: Coping Strategies for Caregivers

Understanding the Caregiver Role

Understanding the caregiver role in the context of diabetes insipidus is crucial for both patients and their families. Caregivers often serve as the primary support system for individuals diagnosed with this condition, which is characterized by an inability to concentrate urine due to insufficient production of antidiuretic hormone (ADH). Their responsibilities extend beyond physical assistance, encompassing emotional support, education about the condition, and coordination of medical care. Understanding the intricacies of this role can significantly enhance the quality of life for patients and help caregivers fulfill their duties more effectively.

The caregiver's role begins with a comprehensive understanding of diabetes insipidus, including its causes and risk factors. Educating themselves about the condition allows caregivers to recognize symptoms, such as excessive thirst and frequent urination, and to understand how these symptoms impact daily life. This knowledge enables caregivers to advocate for their loved ones, ensuring they receive appropriate medical attention and follow-up care. Awareness of the potential complications and long-term effects of diabetes insipidus also equips caregivers to anticipate challenges and seek timely intervention when necessary.

In addition to medical knowledge, caregivers must develop strong communication skills to effectively collaborate with healthcare providers. This collaboration includes sharing observations about the patient's symptoms, medication adherence, and any changes in health status. Caregivers often act as liaisons between patients and medical professionals, ensuring that the patient's concerns and needs are addressed. This role is particularly important during diagnosis and testing, where accurate reporting of symptoms can influence treatment decisions. Caregivers should feel empowered to ask questions and seek clarification about the condition and its management.

Coping with the psychological impact of diabetes insipidus is another vital aspect of the caregiver role. Both patients and caregivers may experience emotional challenges, such as anxiety, stress, or feelings of isolation. Caregivers should be attentive to the emotional well-being of the patient, offering reassurance and understanding. Encouraging open discussions about feelings and concerns can help alleviate some of the emotional burdens associated with the condition. Moreover, caregivers themselves may benefit from seeking support through counseling or support groups, as managing the demands of caregiving can be overwhelming.

Finally, caregivers play a significant role in implementing lifestyle changes and management strategies that enhance the patient's quality of life. This includes helping patients adhere to treatment regimens, encouraging dietary considerations, and supporting the incorporation of healthy habits into daily routines. Caregivers can also assist with monitoring fluid intake and output, which is essential for managing diabetes insipidus effectively. By fostering a supportive environment, caregivers not only help patients navigate their condition but also contribute to a more positive outlook on living with diabetes insipidus.

Communication with Patients

Communication with patients is a critical component in the management of diabetes insipidus. Establishing a clear and open dialogue between healthcare providers and patients can significantly improve understanding and adherence to treatment plans. Patients must feel empowered to express their concerns, ask questions, and share their experiences. This level of communication fosters a supportive environment where patients can better understand their condition and the importance of following medical advice.

When discussing diabetes insipidus, it is essential for healthcare providers to explain the causes and risk factors in a way that is accessible and relatable. Patients should be informed about how the condition affects their body, including the role of the kidneys and the significance of antidiuretic hormone. By breaking down complex medical terminology and using everyday language, healthcare professionals can help patients grasp the underlying mechanisms of their condition. This understanding can alleviate anxiety and create a sense of control over their health.

Diagnosis and testing methods are often a source of confusion for patients. Clear communication about what to expect during diagnostic procedures is vital. Patients should be informed about the types of tests that may be conducted, such as blood tests and water deprivation tests, and the rationale behind them. Providing information about the purpose of these tests and how they will help in developing a treatment plan can reduce apprehension and encourage cooperation. It is equally important to discuss the potential outcomes of these tests to prepare patients for their diagnosis.

Treatment options for diabetes insipidus can vary widely, so it is crucial for patients to have a thorough understanding of their choices. Healthcare providers should explain the different medications available, such as desmopressin, and how they work to manage symptoms. Additionally, discussing lifestyle changes and management strategies can empower patients to take an active role in their care. This includes hydration strategies, dietary considerations, and the importance of regular follow-up appointments. When patients are well-informed about their treatment options, they are more likely to adhere to their prescribed plans and actively participate in their health journey.

Lastly, addressing the psychological impact of living with diabetes insipidus is essential in communication. Patients may experience anxiety, depression, or social withdrawal due to their condition. Healthcare providers should encourage open discussions about these feelings and offer resources for psychological support. It is important for patients to know that they are not alone and that mental health is just as crucial as physical health in managing diabetes insipidus. By fostering a supportive atmosphere where patients can share their struggles and triumphs, healthcare providers can enhance the overall quality of care and improve patients' quality of life.

Self-Care for Caregivers

Self-Care for caregivers of patients with diabetes insipidus is essential for maintaining their own well-being while supporting those they care for. Caregiving can be a demanding role, often leading to physical and emotional exhaustion. It is crucial for caregivers to prioritize their own health to ensure they can provide the best support possible. This begins with recognizing the signs of caregiver burnout, which can include fatigue, irritability, and feelings of being overwhelmed. By acknowledging these feelings early on, caregivers can take proactive steps to address them.

Establishing a self-care routine is vital. This may involve setting aside regular time for activities that promote relaxation and rejuvenation, such as exercise, reading, or engaging in hobbies. Even short breaks throughout the day can significantly impact a caregiver's mental and emotional state. Additionally, caregivers should consider incorporating mindfulness practices, such as meditation or deep-breathing exercises, which can help reduce stress and enhance emotional resilience.

Building a support network is another critical aspect of self-care. Caregivers should seek out friends, family, or support groups who can offer emotional support and understanding. Sharing experiences with others who are in similar situations can provide valuable insights and coping strategies. It is also beneficial for caregivers to communicate their needs with those around them, fostering an environment where they feel comfortable asking for help when needed.

Nutrition and sleep also play a significant role in a caregiver's ability to manage stress and maintain overall health. Caregivers should prioritize a balanced diet that includes a variety of nutrients, as this can improve energy levels and overall well-being. Similarly, ensuring adequate sleep is essential for cognitive function and emotional stability. Caregivers may need to establish a consistent sleep schedule and create a restful environment to enhance their quality of sleep.

Finally, caregivers should not hesitate to seek professional help if they find themselves struggling to cope. Speaking with a counselor or therapist can provide a safe space to process feelings and develop new coping strategies. Ultimately, by prioritizing self-care, caregivers can enhance their ability to support their loved ones with diabetes insipidus while also safeguarding their own health and happiness.

Resources and Support Networks

Resources and support networks play a crucial role in managing diabetes insipidus. Patients often feel overwhelmed by their diagnosis and the accompanying lifestyle changes. Accessing reliable information can empower individuals to make informed decisions about their health. Numerous resources are available, including websites dedicated to endocrine disorders, which offer comprehensive insights into the causes, symptoms, and management of diabetes insipidus. Organizations such as the National Institute of Diabetes and Digestive and Kidney Diseases provide educational materials that can help patients better understand their condition and navigate their treatment options.

Support networks can significantly enhance the quality of life for individuals living with diabetes insipidus. Local support groups, whether in-person or online, enable patients to connect with others facing similar challenges. These groups provide a platform for sharing experiences, coping strategies, and emotional support. Additionally, virtual communities and forums can offer a wealth of knowledge from individuals who have managed diabetes insipidus for years, fostering a sense of belonging and reducing feelings of isolation.

Healthcare professionals are invaluable resources in the management of diabetes insipidus. Patients should not hesitate to reach out to endocrinologists, nurses, and dietitians who specialize in this area. These professionals can provide tailored advice, help in understanding treatment options, and assist in the development of personalized management plans. Regular consultations with healthcare providers are essential for monitoring the condition, making necessary adjustments to treatment, and addressing any emerging concerns.

Educational workshops and seminars can also serve as effective support avenues. Many hospitals and health organizations offer programs aimed at educating patients and their families about diabetes insipidus. Topics may include understanding the underlying causes, recognizing symptoms, and exploring lifestyle modifications. Engaging in these educational opportunities not only equips patients with valuable knowledge but also fosters a collaborative approach to managing their health.

Lastly, mental health resources should not be overlooked. The psychological impact of living with a chronic condition like diabetes insipidus can be significant. Counseling and therapy services can help patients deal with the emotional challenges associated with their diagnosis. Support from mental health professionals can assist in developing coping mechanisms and improving overall well-being. By utilizing a combination of these resources and support networks, patients can enhance their ability to manage diabetes insipidus effectively.